LIFESTYLE CHANGE

Powerful Lessons in Personal Improvement

Nash Jocic

LIFESTYLE CHANGE
Powerful Lessons in Personal Improvement

Nash Jocic

Ultimate Shape Limited

London 2009

This edition published 2009 in Great Britain by
Ultimate Shape Limited
PO BOX 497 48
London
N20 0SJ

A catalogue record for this book is available from the British Library.

FIRST EDITION

Published in the United Kingdom

ISBN 978-0-9562598-1-3

Disclaimer:

This book is NOT intended to replace in any way the services of a physician, or as a
treatment or prevention for diseases, or an alternative to professional medical advice.
This book is a review of the author's own experience from the fields of lifestyle,
nutrition and resistance training and is presented for informational purposes and to
increase awareness of the importance of living a healthy lifestyle.

To my dear parents, Nada and Mile Jocic and
my aunt Beba, with love and respect.

Contents

Who Are We?

From the very beginning of our existence, humans have continually been exposed to different living environments. Some were relaxed and easy, but most were very harsh and difficult. Throughout human evolution our constantly changing environment has been the most significant factor in the creation of our lifestyle. Millions of years of adaptation to this changing environment produced lifestyles which had a profound effect on our physiology. All our bodily systems (skeletal, muscular, digestive, vascular and others) were developed through physical and mental activities brought about by our need to survive.

The development of agriculture made human life much easier and resulted in a huge expansion of the world's population. Manufacturing and later on industrialisation, with their unprecedented technological advancement, once again dramatically changed our living environment. The resulting lifestyle was much less challenging and more secure and comfortable, but while it offered huge benefits, at the same time it introduced previously unknown physical and mental conditions.

Suddenly humans no longer needed to rely upon their physical activities as much as they had in the past. Strength, speed, agility and endurance were no longer as essential to our survival as before. At the same time, in the post-industrial world our bodily systems started encountering pressures that had not existed before.

Our sedentary lifestyles and the contamination of basic elements of survival such as water, air and food, have had a huge impact on our physiology.

Despite our achievements in prolonging life and fighting illness with the aid of technology, we appear to have actually *diminished* the capability of our bodily systems to deal with the environment. Technological progress has accomplished a great deal, but there are other, much more efficient and beneficial ways in which we can improve our health and longevity. Following the natural order of life, we can maintain good health and attain quality of life that pushes the boundaries of our genetic limitations.

In biological terms, natural selection has almost disappeared in modern humans, despite having been a valid principle for hundreds of thousands of years. Mental awareness, quick reaction times, strength, stamina, the ability to make fast decisions – these were much more important for survival in the daily lives of our ancestors than they are for us today.

Instinct, the invisible hand that had guided so many aspects of our existence, has lost precedence to our newly-found reliance upon skill and technology. We used to *sense* danger; we relied upon our instincts to get the appreciation and respect of others, to choose a partner, reproduce, trust a friend, to protect and help others. Now, when our instincts stir inside us, suggesting a solution, we often do not know what to do with these feelings. We instead call upon our intellect alone to help us, suppressing those instincts and burying them deep inside, where we think they belong. This practice is not as innocent as it may seem. This pattern of denying instinctive feelings is the source of many mental and physical problems. Although physiologically and mentally we are still very similar to our ancestors of 150.000 years ago, we now live in a very different environment. We have distanced ourselves from Mother Nature more than ever before. We no longer like food in its natural state because it is 'boring'. We like our modern, man-manipulated food because it tastes 'better'. We do not use our naturally evolved physiques as the nature intended because we consider ourselves to be an 'intellectual' species. Consequently, we involve ourselves daily in pursuits that require little or no physical activity.

At the same time, this new lifestyle introduces a great deal of stress into our lives. In the last 30 years we have witnessed dramatic changes in our lifestyle. Technological progress has pushed our way of life into previously unknown and completely unexpected directions. We have never lived our lives at such a fast pace and the amount of daily stress has never been higher; we have never experienced having so many responsibilities and so much pressure, and at the same time we have never nourished our bodies as inadequately as we do today.

Our system of values has also undergone radical change. Things that had been of the utmost importance in the past, such as marriage, family and friendships, have in modern times dropped down on our list of priorities. Today we prefer to be single (as that helps us deal with work overload) and we don't seek commitments. Nowadays we back away from social responsibilities, we delay pregnancies until they become almost impossible, and we value material over intellectual and spiritual wealth.

Commenting on the new system of values inevitably generates arguments for and against. Values are not absolute in themselves, they change in different times and they vary in different cultures. However, being able to draw on new values and to take advantage of them is certainly very important to us. This is because we can strive to evolve our system of values to become of maximum assistance to us, as individuals and as a species. Therefore, we can ask ourselves: "Do we benefit in all the ways possible from our contemporary system of values? Do we really live a better life as a result of the choice of lifestyle that modern man has made?"

Our new system of values and modern lifestyle have undoubtedly helped the industrialised world to move forward and grow. We do have stronger economies, we do produce bigger GDP and we are economically better off and able to help others. We invest more in science, research, education and health care. But are we really doing so well? No, we are not.

The biggest problem facing us today is that the lifestyle we have adopted is actually killing us, one by one. Its effect on our physical wellbeing means that we are dying by the thousands from the ailments that had never existed before. Terminal or serious physical illnesses, as well as new kinds of disabilities and mental disorders are today commonplace. The level of cardiovascular disease is constantly rising, we have more respiratory problems than ever before and there is a huge increase in incidence of obesity, diabetes, cancers and allergies. The list goes on.

So what are we doing wrong? We try our best, we work hard to achieve greater security, we value work above everything else, we constantly strive for more and yet most of us continue to experience a deluge of heath problems. Difficulties in moving, feeling sick, tiring quickly, fainting, losing energy, getting weak and depressed - the list of modern-day symptoms seems endless. Our new reality is that we are not able to work any more! We cannot function at our peak level and thus we lose the power and respect we worked so hard to achieve and experience a decline in our life quality. Our system of values starts drifting away from us, until we finally lose sight of it altogether. We cannot rely on it any more. We find ourselves on the outside, we don't fit in any more and we feel abandoned and betrayed.

Is this the only possible outcome for a life of ignorance and misunderstanding? Is there anything we can do to change this situation, or even to prevent it? Can we work hard and enjoy the benefits of our modern technology and still be healthy and prosperous? Is there light at the end of the tunnel?

The answer lies in changing our lifestyle; getting back to what we were in the first place - complex physical as well as intellectual and spiritual beings. We cannot afford to ignore any element of our existence. There are ways in which modern society can be adapted to allow us to perform with even greater efficiency and live happier and healthier lives.

The Importance of Health

"He who has health has hope; he who has hope has everything."
- Arabian proverb

*"Health is the greatest of all possessions, a pale
cobbler is better than a sick king."*
- Isaac Bickerstaff

According to the World Health Organisation, health is 'a complete state of physical, mental and social well-being, not just the absence of disease'. This definition clearly describes health as concerning both our physical and emotional well-being.

Being physically healthy means that your body is functioning properly, free of pain, discomfort or lack of capabilities. Common causes of ill health include injuries, disease, poor diet, stress, old age and genetic predisposition.

Being emotionally and mentally healthy means that your mind and emotions function as they should, free of anxiety, depression or other malfunctions. Common causes of mental ill health include physical disease, stress, genetic predisposition and mental abuse.

Being physically healthy is of utmost importance for life. Being ill or not feeling well significantly affects your ability to work and perform well. Emotional well-being is just as important, as suffering stress, depression, anxiety or other mental and emotional ailments affects both our physical health and our ability to work. Clearly, feeling physically and mentally healthy makes you much more productive, as well as more contented.

Work is only one of the many components of life. We must be able to enjoy all its other aspects in order to achieve longevity, productivity and a fulfilling existence. Taking interest in our physical well-being enables us to expand our knowledge and skills, to perform well and gain respect of our employers, colleagues and peers. On a more personal level, if we are in good physical and mental health, our family and friends enjoy our company more, we are able to take better care of them and help them prosper in their lives.

Good health is the most significant asset our lives provide for us, but also our biggest responsibility. Ultimately, it is up to all of us to take responsibility for ourselves, our family, friends and people in our work and social environment. Good health cannot be taken for granted. We have to be prepared to make positive efforts to achieve, support and maintain good health for the sake of our own happiness, and the happiness of those around us.

> *"Health is ability to work and to love."*
> - Freud

Our Living Environment

Throughout the course of our evolution our living environment has been the most powerful factor affecting our lifestyle. External factors continually exert their influence, shaping and altering our inner fabric and mental structure. Until the onset of the industrialisation, our living conditions were extremely difficult and there were rarely long periods of security, prosperity and the abundance of food. Human beings were engaged in a constant struggle with environmental changes and completely preoccupied with gathering food, hunting and protecting themselves and their family group. The daily fight for survival involved strenuous physical work as well as deep mental engagement.

With the discovery of agriculture, some 10.000 years ago, we were able to speed up the process of evolution. Instead of only hunting and gathering, we started manipulating the world around us in a much more profound way. As agriculture brought about a worldwide increase in human population, natural resources became scarce and this led to endless wars, conflicts and destruction. On the other hand, population growth and scarcity of natural resources also had the effect of forcing humans to start changing the environment they live in rather than simply adapting to it.

Nature has never granted us anything for free. Every advancement in the quality of our lives had to be earned. It took millions of years of trial and error to get to where we are today. As humanity evolved into a superior species, a variety of cultures emerged in different parts of the world. They all had the same aim – to enhance the quality of life for those living within them. Despite being genetically and physiologically identical, people from different cultures possessed different levels of knowledge and consequently developed divergent lifestyles. Values that were held in high regard in some civilisations were not so highly regarded in others. Priorities that drove the politics and the economies of certain cultures did not mean much to others. Our intellectual achievement may have been disparate, but we were still all members of the human race, identical in our physiologies and with the same reactions to the outside factors. Cultural blindness (viewing world events through the limited set of values and norms learned in one's own culture) has clearly created a history of sharp divisions and conflicts among the peoples of the world.

Diverse cultures gave rise to different religions which became a potent new source of influence that further deepened the differences within humanity. People started believing in a variety of divine creators, until major civilisations finally settled in their belief in a single creator, who alone grants us the opportunity to exist in our human form. But although people from around the world believed in the divine, they couldn't agree which one was the true god. Different religions were spreading different messages, following different prophets and offering different values. And yet, despite all these differences, we were still members of the same species, regardless of the part of the world we came from.

Diverse cultures with their different religions generated different sets of traditions and customs around the globe. Customs are patterns of behaviour that have, over time and trough repetition, become inherent in a given culture, fixed and effortlessly carried out. Unsurprisingly, customs and traditions are never questioned; we see them as intrinsic to our societies. We are raised to believe that they are indisputable and infallible. But, are they? We know from experience, for example, that there are many conditions and diseases that are common in certain cultures, while in others some other ailments are more pervasive. It is clear that a strong attachment to and a large prevalence of habitual behaviour patterns does not necessarily benefit the cultures that generate and follow them. These habitual behaviour patterns may have been of great importance in the developing stages of human societies, but they have undeservedly continued to affect the rules of life in modern times.

If we view the individual as a citizen of the world, regardless of his or her culture, religion and race, we realise that all the differences in the world put together cannot defy global prosperity. We can see new evidence of this every day. Some of the most traditional cultures in the world which have been closed to the outside world for thousands of years are opening up, welcoming different values, and benefiting greatly from this new openness. People from different races, cultures and religions are increasingly mixing and living together united by the same goal – a better quality of life and greater prosperity.

The world is once again becoming what it always has been in its essence – a unified entity. Instead of the cultural and religious differences separating us, we are achieving increasing unity, driven by scientific understanding and a logical approach to solving problems. The reality of the modern world is that we are becoming increasingly receptive to the fact that we are all ultimately the same, with identical responses to both beneficial and harmful external factors. We are slowly realising that we have to stand together and act as a global entity if we hope to solve the problems facing us today and to prosper.

Commitment to work

A single principle that unites us in today's world is our commitment to work. We all work for more or less the same reasons – to support ourselves, our families, to achieve status or dominance within the group, to feel secure. Motives can vary to some extent, but the need to work is the same for all of us - we have to work in order to achieve good-quality lives.

In today's world our places of work have become much more than somewhere to trade our skills for money. Work has become a place where we live socially, a platform that allows us to express many of the characteristics that make us human – the need to compete, dominate, attract, persuade, give and receive. We all expect to be respected and appreciated at work, we all want to contribute as much as possible and be a part of a successful organisation. We continually strive to improve.

We develop a hierarchy of priorities in our lives almost instinctively. Our choice is driven by cultural values, the times we live in and peer pressure. Selecting a wrong sequence of priorities frequently results in the different problems we experience in the areas of our physical and mental health. We often neglect the most essential elements for our survival and watch them move down our list of priorities because we believe that certain other things are more important. A correct selection and sequence of priorities is affirmed only through a life that progresses effortlessly, without major difficulties.

All the factors mentioned so far help us to create our own lifestyle. A lifestyle may be understood as the way in which we live our lives: the way we eat, communicate, select priorities, the way we take care of ourselves and others, what we believe, how we give and receive, and how we love and hate.

So we really need to ask ourselves the following question: "Is my lifestyle good enough, is it helping me to be happier, more prosperous and responsible, or is there something that needs to change in order to allow me to improve my life?"

Let's look at an average day in our lives. More often than not we wake up feeling quite unhappy and actually rather tired, and we have to force ourselves out of bed. We rush to the kitchen to make the 'revitalising' brew of strong coffee or tea before we get dressed for work in work clothes that we loathe. Some of us have to take children to school, which means waking them up, washing, dressing and feeding them, preparing lunch boxes, all the while trying our utmost to be the perfect parent. Some children need us to humour them or tell them a story to prepare them for the day. Running late, you finally deliver them to school, and then you are free. Free to do what? Go to work! As if all the effort spent just getting to that point was not enough!

But, there you are; at least you managed to find a parking space quickly – your lucky day! You walk to the office with the day already planned out in detail. You have your targets and you know what you have to do to achieve them. At least that's what you think. You soon discover that there are a few obstacles in the way. Your other colleagues, for example, are striving towards the same targets, and there's your boss who cares only for success, results and profit. In effect, you must compete with your colleagues, which is a far cry from all the motivational talk about teamwork. But you have no choice. Whether you are successful at work or not affects not just you, but your family as well. You constantly worry about having to buy a new house, mounting school fees, bills that keep piling up... It's very hard to perform well in the work environment if you have the weight of the world on your shoulders!

After a while of trying to work while preoccupied with the worries of your everyday life, you get that annoying spasm in your abdomen. You have felt the same twitch for several weeks now. Or is it several months? Have you been trying to ignore it? Could it be that you are avoiding the fact that something might be the matter with you? You probably forgot to eat this morning, and your first meal of the day was at 1pm, consisting of either a sandwich, hamburger or pizza. It has probably been some time since you had some fruit and vegetables. Can you even remember the last time you eat together with your family?

You somehow manage to get through the first part of the day, fuelled by several cups of coffee, some biscuits and your unwholesome lunch in the nondescript staff canteen. The rest of the time you spend sitting at your desk and staring at the computer. Finally you make it to the end of your working day. As you try to stand up from your chair your lower back suddenly gives out, and you find yourself unable to move! The old lower back problem has come back to haunt you. It's been troubling you for years. And when was the last time you went to the gym? Can you even recall the last time you took some exercise? It now becomes painfully obvious that some changes must be made or else you must be prepared to suffer the consequences.

You arrive home exhausted and stressed but you feel you must hide that from your partner and children. By pretending that everything is all right you are actually piling more stress on top of all the pressure you have accumulated through the day. You are constantly and agonisingly aware that your family heavily depend upon you for security and prosperity. It is unquestionable that, in order to deliver all that is expected, you have to be in great mental and physical shape. Are you?

If you recognise aspects of your own life in any of the above, you can take a little comfort in the fact that you are not alone - there are millions of people around the world who lead similar lives, burdened by the same responsibilities and problems as you. Should this really make you feel better? I'm afraid not. Your poor lifestyle has to be changed. You have to assume full responsibility for yourself and for your family and people that matter to you. Neglecting a problem you know about is worse than not knowing you have one. You cannot afford to ignore the signs - if something is not right, you must fix it. And you must start the process of change immediately, as soon as you realise you have a problem. Putting it off will not help. The longer you wait, the more the situation will deteriorate. So, is there a way to change this pattern, this daily cycle we are trapped in which offers such a bleak future? Yes, there is.

Consequences of a Poor Lifestyle

In recent times life has changed dramatically for all of us. We are witnessing the unprecedented rise in the world population, increased production of goods, rapid movement of capital, huge changes in technology and information delivery, and increased competition in the work place and world markets. We live our lives at a faster pace, with more duties and responsibilities. All of these changes significantly affect the lifestyle of the workforce of today.

In today's terms, our unrelenting desire for a better life ultimately translates into earning more money. Money is identified with freedom, power and better quality of life. Any person who has made 'enough' money knows, however, that money alone does not solve all our problems. As long as money is considered just a tool, a means by which we reach for the things that are beneficial to us, everything is achievable. Once money becomes a goal in itself, horizons close. Increases in wealth and technological progress have also created misery for many people, who, caught in the midst of the merciless race of life forget to think about their health, fitness, and proper nutrition. Once essential elements of our lives, these crucial prerogatives have become marginalised in today's fast-moving society. But health, fitness and proper diet have never lost their place in terms of contributing to our overall quality of life. For people who understand these lifestyle principles and practice them in the way they deserve to be practised, the quality of life will remain high. Those who ignore or neglect them will inevitably face serious consequences that manifest themselves in deteriorating health, lack of motivation, loss of satisfaction, depression, etc.

In addition, people are becoming less social nowadays, they see their friends less frequently and even family members feel like strangers for many of people. We seem less able to love, to care about ourselves, we commit less often and we limit our freedom, energy and creativity. But what for?

At the start of every person's story we usually find the same prologue – a struggle for recognition, approval, money and/or progress. The trouble is that the prologue, keeping up the same struggle, seems to last forever, although perhaps on different levels. That constant effort to stay on top frequently deprives us of our basic instinctive feelings, those intuitive clues that help us to recognise who we can trust, what food is right for us, and how to select physical activities that will make us stronger and more resistant to every-day pressures. In many ways we seem to have lost a connection with our key instinct, that of survival. If this instinct were still strong in us we would not harm ourselves as we do, essentially diminishing our chances of a long and fruitful existence by consistently living the wrong lifestyle.

Boundaries of age have been established in order to keep us happier in the later stages of our lives, when we realise that life slows down in time. Milestones of age are there to remind us that we should 'age with dignity'. You don't have to accept that point of view, however. Perhaps like me, you'd rather live with dignity than age with dignity. Who is to say where the boundary point is? At which stage, during which year, on which particular day of life do we start aging? From my own experience, and from the experience of my clients who have been following the lifestyle advice proposed here, I can categorically state that age boundaries can be dramatically moved. I have seen clients in their sixties perform to a level that people in their twenties can only dream about! There is no magic – what I teach has been proven to work for thousands of people around the globe. If you set your mind correctly and you have a strong desire to live healthily and improve the quality of your life, you will achieve your goal.

Life can slow down at any point in time, as soon as you decide it should. If what you want is to feel continuously tired, out of shape, depressed, unhappy, negative and against everything and everybody, you don't have to wait to get to a certain age! You can achieve that at any time, in fact it will not take a great deal of effort or enthusiasm. If that is what you expect and strive for, you can a achieve it easily. You can slow down in your twenties, thirties, or whenever you decide it is time to grow old. This slowing down process is what I call aging.

But you can decide not to slow down. You certainly won't if you believe you have something to offer to yourself and to others. So,

what is this idea of slowing down all about? Take a look at the
great success stories in our midst – great composers, scientists,
artists, writers, actors, politicians and philosophers. They all live
their lives to the full, because they constantly give more of themselves to others. They have something within themselves to share
with others and that is why they are able to keep giving and forget
about slowing down. We have all met individuals in their sixties
and seventies who simply refuse to act old, and instead offer so
much motivation and energy to those around them that they are
continuously gaining deeper knowledge and understanding. And
this is possible simply because such people reject the idea of
slowing down. In their lives, negligence and ignorance have been
overcome by expression and giving. This is what I see as the only
way forward for all humanity. Life should be understood as an opportunity to evolve, mature and then give to others.

I have always understood life as an opportunity to achieve something, something for myself that will make me a dignified person
in the community. Something that would enable me to stand up
and say what I think and have enough credibility so that others
listen to what I have to say. I wanted my ideas to be understood
and applied in order to improve the quality of life for others. I
strived to become someone who is able to listen to others and understand their approaches, teachings, experiences and problems.
And also to be an equal player in the arena of life.

In my search for the right way of living a good lifestyle, I have come to realise that most of our problems arise from a mixed-up order of accomplishments. In this life, if we are to have undisrupted intellectual and moral progress to maturity, we must develop in a certain order. In the process of development, only a healthy and capable physical body can serve as the vehicle which will propel us from the bottom to the top. Besides, unless we adopt a correct lifestyle to help us achieve a healthy body we cannot expect to have enough time and life-force to provide for our intellectual and spiritual maturity anyway.

Our body is our temple, the only one we have and it should be the starting point in our preparations for the race of life. The more we take care of the body, the better position we can expect to secure. Our emotional, social, parental and many other aspects of life depend directly on the way our physical being develops. If we neglect our physical ethos, many other aspects of our life will inevitably suffer.

Among the common problems created by the overwhelming expectations of our increasingly competitive economies and our struggle to survive in that world, there are three that, from my point of view, deserve most attention. These three are: Stress, Inactivity and Diet.

Stress

Generally, we can describe stress as any force that, when applied to a system, causes significant modification, usually connoting the modification to be in a form of deformation or distortion. The term is used with respect to physical, psychological and social forces and pressures.

Types of Stress

There are four main types of stress that we can experience: eustress, distress, hyperstress and hypostress.

Eustress – eustress is a positive, short-term stress, which provides us with instant strength. Eustress arises when motivation and inspiration are heightened, at the point of increased physical activity, enthusiasm and creativity.

Distress – distress is a negative stress that creates feelings of discomfort or anxiety and there are two types: acute and chronic. Acute distress is intense and it arises and disappears quickly. Chronic distress is a prolonged state that can go on for weeks, months or even years. Chronic distress is the type of stress that is of great interest to us here.

Hyperstress – hyperstress occurs when an individual is pushed beyond what he or she can handle. Hyper stress results from being overloaded or overworked. When someone is hyperstressed, even little things can trigger a strong emotional response.

Hypostress – hypostress is the opposite of hyperstress. Hypostress occurs when an individual is bored or unchallenged. People who experience hypostress are often restless and uninspired.

Causes of Stress

There are three categories of causes of stress – general causes, life causes and work-related causes.

1) General causes:

Threats – threats encompass physical, social, financial and emotional threats. Even a threat that is only perceived can make a person feel stressed. Being unable to respond to a threat can cause loss of control, which invariably makes the situation worse.

Fear – threats provoke fear, which leads to stress. Fear leads us to imagine frightening outcomes, the real source of stress.

Uncertainty – when we are not certain about our situation we are unable to predict what will happen, and that makes us feel that we are not in control. This often leads to the feelings of fear and imminent danger.

2) Life causes:

- Death: of a spouse, member of the family, friend
- Health: injury, illness, pregnancy
- Crime: sexual molestation, mugging, burglary
- Self-abuse: drug abuse, alcoholism, self-harm
- Family change: marriage, separation, divorce
- Sexual problems: lack of sexual relationship, maintaining good sexual relationship
- Physical changes: lack of sleep, exhaustion, aging
- Money: having it, the lack of it, investing it, pension
- Work: job security, relationship with colleagues and managers, change in working hours

3.) The UK Health and Safety Executive lists six key work-related stress factors:

- Job demands
- The control staff have over how they do their work
- The support they receive from colleagues and superiors
- The relationship with colleagues
- Whether or not they understand their roles and responsibilities
- How far the company consults staff over workplace changes

Other work-related stress factors include:

- Sickness, absence
- Poor communication between teams
- Bullying
- Value of one's contribution
- Lack of clarity of one's roles and responsibilities
- Working long hours
- One-off incidents
- Uncomfortable workplace

Symptoms of Stress

Although stress can be experienced in all areas of life, work-related stress is the most common cause of sickness absence across the industries, resulting in billions lost by businesses every year.

The most common symptoms of stress are:

- High blood pressure
- Heart conditions
- Muscle catabolism
- Fatigue
- Digestion changes
- Ulcers
- Loss of sexual drive
- Sleep pattern changes

- Headaches
- Anxiety
- Depression
- Hormonal imbalance
- Weakened immunity
- Infections
- Back and neck pains
- Alcoholism
- Smoking
- Anorexia
- Bulimia
- Lack of concentration
- Memory lapses
- Confusion
- Panic attacks

It is apparent from the long list of the consequences of stress that not a single body system is spared from its effects. All the body systems: skeletal, muscular, cardiovascular, digestive, nervous and endocrine, as well as the body's immunity are dramatically affected by stress.

Inactivity

Inactivity causes many of our physical and mental problems. Representing a drastic rejection of the basic requirements of human anatomy and physiology, inactivity is a completely unnatural state for both our physical and mental being. There are over 600 muscles in the human body, and they were unquestionably not designed to remain inactive day in, day out, week after week, year after year. Just like our other supportive systems such as cardiovascular, respiratory or endocrine, muscular system needs to be engaged on a daily basis in order to perform optimally. All of these systems have to be stimulated regularly and sufficiently in order to perform with maximum efficiency and provide us with strength, stamina, good health and mental power.

Let's take a look at some of the bodily systems most adversely affected by inactivity:

Skeletal system – with inactivity, the skeletal system will weaken and deform through being insufficiently utilized by a weak and disproportionately developed muscular system .

Muscular system – the muscular system provides stimulus and impetus for optimal performance of all other systems. Through inactivity it is denied its own nature. If muscles remain inactive, they will atrophy and lead to premature aging of other supporting systems (i.e. cardiovascular, respiratory, endocrine).

Cardiovascular system – the heart, arteries, veins and capillaries are all adversely affected by inactivity, which causes cholesterol deposits in the arteries, weakening of the heart muscle, high blood pressure and poor circulation. The more advanced illnesses of the cardiovascular system are also very common in people who adopt inactive lifestyles.

Endocrine system – life-boosting hormones such as testosterone and growth hormone reach their optimum levels only in physically active individuals. The positive impact they have on cardiovascular health, bone density, metabolism, insulin sensitivity, body-fat levels, libido and fertility, is well established. The point at which we start to age, in a sense of experiencing the diminishing in our capabilities, coincides with the decrease in the production and secretion of testosterone and growth hormone. It is very common for the production of both these hormones to diminish in the last fifty years of life, mainly due to physical inactivity. There are millions of people around the world suffering from problems caused by hormonal deficiency or imbalance.

Immune system – working in balance with other bodily systems, the immune system responds promptly to the condition of other systems. If just one of them runs into difficulties and slows down, that will have an immediate effect on the immune system. If it is to defend the body from the different bacteria and viruses that are in or around us all the time, the immune system must function efficiently. Deficiency in our immune system is one of the most common reasons why we are so susceptible to illness. An overstretched immune system will never offer optimal protection from common acute and chronic diseases. Inactivity is one of the major causes of an overstretched and weakened immune system.

Mental state – Our mental state reflects our physical health, which, it is commonly accepted, is directly influenced by everyday activity. Depression and anxiety are the most common psychological consequences of inactivity. The interaction between our physical and mental states of being is of crucial importance because these two systems influence each other constantly. A healthy physical state will deliver a healthy mental state. A healthy mental state will always enhance physical efficiency. A weakened and troubled physical body will never lead to a strong and healthy mental state.

Consequences of Inactivity

- Increased risk of dying prematurely
- Increased risk of developing heart disease
- Increased risk of developing diabetes
- High blood pressure
- Increased risk of developing colon cancer

- Depression and anxiety
- Obesity
- Hormonal imbalance
- Aches and pains
- Lower back problems
- Neck problems
- Weak bones and joints
- Weak muscles and connective tissues
- Decreased mobility
- Decreased psychological well-being

Poor Diet

Modern lifestyle has presented us with another major setback: inappropriate diet. Influenced by the fast pace of life, diverging cultural habits, poor selection of priorities in life and a lack of proper information, we are left with very few options when it comes to nutrition. With limited free time, which is a prevalent feature of our modern lifestyle, food doesn't stand a chance of regaining its rightful place and receiving the attention it deserves. We see food as a quick fix, never as something essential that deserves time and attention in terms of its selection, preparation and consumption. By today's standards, food has to be cheap, tasty, pre-prepared and readily available. We choose which food to select and consume based on these requirements. This choice is clearly wrong. Nothing but high-quality, properly selected and combined food – which takes time to prepare and enjoy – should be of human interest. None of us can afford to compromise our health.

Our bodies always find a way of dealing with poor eating habits, but not without consequences. All bodily systems suffer as a result of inadequate diet, some of them more, some less. Some will give up sooner, some later, but they will all inevitably respond in undesirable ways.

Another significant problem is that we eat far too much. Food which is readily available, any place and at any time, is extremely difficult to resist! Over the last fifty years we have adopted alarmingly unnatural eating patterns. We eat at the prescribed times, but we also snack between our meals, so we are actually eating all day long. Most of the food we consume is very dry, dense in calories and full of ingredients that our digestive systems hardly recognise and have trouble digesting. The major macronutrients in our daily diet are carbohydrates and fats, which makes every meal a proper caloric bomb! The number of calories we consume in a single meal often exceeds the number of calories we need for the whole day. In our modern industrialised world we no longer eat to satisfy hunger, because we are hardly ever properly hungry any more. We eat to feel full, and as a consequence of that, we overeat. Our improper diets are responsible for all of our chronic diseases today including cancer, diabetes, cardiovascular disease, allergies, tooth decay, and many more.

In order to determine what the right diet is, we need to take a look at how we nourished ourselves in the course of human history. We should pay particular attention to the periods in human evolution in which chronic diseases appear to have been non-existent. What was the diet that provided humanity with vigorous strength and good health? What were we eating 15.000 years ago that resulted in the recently found skeletons from that period showing perfect bone and dental development, completely free of deformities or decay? And this excellent state of health of those teeth, for example, was achieved without the benefit of toothpaste, tooth brushes, fluoride tablets or dentists! The answers to our question about the right diet may lie in our past eating habits.

Consequences of Poor Diet

Scientific research has clearly demonstrated that what and how much we eat profoundly affects our growth, development, process of aging and the ability to enjoy life to the full.   Dietary intake and the lack of exercise are linked to increased risks of developing common chronic diseases that are both disabling and life-threatening. Here are just some of the consequences of a poor diet that we face today:

*   Diabetes
*   Heart disease
*   Stroke
*   Cancer
*   High blood pressure
*   Tooth decay
*   Ulcers
*   Gastritis
*   Infections
*   Poor memory
*   Anorexia
*   Bulimia

- Osteoporosis
- Pulmonary disease
- Dry skin
- Weak nails and hearing loss
- Adult acne

Health Statistics Related to Stress, Inactivity and Poor Diet

In this chapter we will look at some health statistics relevant to our subject, including some shocking figures obtained from US and UK medical sources. The data clearly shows the consequences of adopting the wrong kind of lifestyle, mainly through physical inactivity and improper diet. The statistics are only useful if they help to raise awareness and illustrate just how essential proper physical engagement and healthy eating habits are for all our systems.

The figures presented here are a product of illnesses and diseases that are largely self-inflicted. I am of the view that, as a society, our general good health depends on each and every individual taking responsibility for their own well-being. Health is not an advantage available only to a privileged few; it is a natural condition, within everyone's reach, that comes as a result of adopting a natural lifestyle. By simply following the requirements of nature and fulfilling our anatomical and physiological needs through proficient physical activity and skilled nutrition, we can regain what has been a human privilege from the start - good health. The statistics are meaningless in themselves, but when put in the context of changes we can make, if we take them as a stimulus and a wake-up call, they assume great significance. Let's take a look at some of them.

Obesity

- 46 percent of men in The UK are classified as overweight.
- 32 percent of women in The UK are classified as overweight.
- 21 percent of men are classified as obese in The UK.
- 23 percent of women are classified as obese in The UK.
- The percentage of adults who are classified as obese has doubled since the mid 1980s.
- Obesity in children under 11 increased from 9.9 percent in 1995 to 13.7 percent in 2003.
- In the UK, one in four children between the ages of 11 and 15 are classified as overweight or obese.
- 8.5 percent of six year-olds and 15 percent of 15 year-olds are classified as obese.
- In 2000, 27 percent of girls between the ages of 2 and 19 were classified as overweight compared to 20 percent of boys of the same age. In the same year, 7 percent of girls were classified as obese, compared to 5 percent of boys.

Cardiovascular Disease (CVD)

- Heart and circulatory disease are UK's biggest killers. In 2002, CVD caused 39 percent of deaths and killed just under 238 .000 people in the UK.
- CVD claimed 869.724 lives in the US in 2004.
- US estimate for 2005 predicted that 80.7 million people would be infected by one or more forms of CVD, 73 million

people would suffer high blood pressure, 16 million people would get coronary heart disease, 5.8 million people would have a stroke and 5.3 million people would suffer heart failure.

Coronary heart disease (CHD)

- Coronary heart disease is the most common cause of premature death among people who are obese. The National Audit Office (NAO) estimates that obesity caused close to 28.000 heart attacks and 750.000 cases of hypertension in the UK in 1998.
- Coronary heart disease in average kills 110 .000 people in the UK every year.
- More than 1.4 million people suffer from angina.
- 275 .000 people have heart attacks every year in the UK.
- Key lifestyle risk factors for CHD include smoking, poor diet and lack of exercise.
- 10 million people in the UK smoke.

Diabetes

- 2.35 million people have diabetes in the UK.
- Type 2 diabetes is closely related to obesity. Obese women are 12 times more likely to develop type 2 diabetes than women of healthy weight. The NAO estimates that obesity was the direct cause of more than 250.000 cases of type 2 diabetes in the UK in 1998.

Osteoporosis

- In the UK, one in two women and one in five men over the age of 50 have osteoporosis.
- In the US, osteoporosis is a major threat to public health with an estimated 44 million sufferers, or 55 percent of people who are aged 50 or older.
- 80 percent of sufferers are women.
- Osteoporosis accounts for 70 percent of all bone fractures for people over 45 in the US.
- There are 1.5 million fractures due to osteoporosis every year in the US.
- Osteoarthritis and back pain are often associated with obesity.

Cancer

- Obesity increases the risk of colon cancer in both men and women nearly threefold.

Lifestyle Change

We have every right to feel proud of our accomplishments because it has taken us a great deal of courage, effort, wisdom and passion to get where we are today. Through millennia of trial and error we have managed to survive as a species, sustain life, improve living conditions and wrestle with the powers of nature with great success. As a civilisation we have made giant steps forward, and we continue to progress in spite of the obstacles standing in our way, seemingly getting bigger and more difficult to overcome all the time.

In modern times we are becoming victims of our own nature. The force that propels us forward is sometimes too strong and too fast and it can itself become a cause of various problems. We constantly want more, we expect better, we want it faster and for longer. It seems that our appetite for life has never been more voracious. And it looks like there is nothing standing in the way of our insatiable greed and relentless desire for advancement. It would be difficult, indeed impossible, to attempt to slow the wheel of history that has gathered such speed. So, if we cannot change the world we live in, can we at least try to adapt to a faster pace of life, with less effort and suffering on our part? Is there anything left for us to change? Is it possible for us to be healthier, happier, more motivated and creative? Can we help ourselves become still more focused and better able to cope with work-related stress?

Health and prosperity are not only meant to be experienced by a privileged few, everyone is entitled to them. As long as we all act responsibly towards ourselves and the people around us, there is a real possibility of attaining both. There are changes we can make to bring ourselves into a new relationship with the world around us. It is possible to achieve better health, more vigour, enthusiasm, prosperity and happiness by making some simple, but crucial lifestyle changes.

Although we will touch upon all the areas relevant to improving our lifestyles, we will pay particular attention to those we consider most neglected in our lives - physical activity through exercise and nutrition through healthy diet.

Our areas of interest fall into the following categories:

1) Information
2) Motivation
3) Action
4) Physical activity through exercise
5) Nutrition through healthy diet

Information

Our intellectual development gets into full flow the moment we are born. Our intellect starts developing rapidly, influenced by the first impressions we receive: the images of our parents and siblings and the sounds we hear in the form of language and music. Information received through the senses helps us to generate our first responses to the world around us and to start communicating, acquiring knowledge and maturing into different characters and personalities. Intellect reaches maturity much later in life, through learning, reading and experiencing life.

From very early on, we are bombarded with information emanating from many different fields of human activity. Much of it is good, constructive information that makes us more capable of achieving our goals in life, but there is also a huge amount of superfluous information that we absorb in the form of advertising, trivial books, bad TV, tabloid press, cheap art and design, and a host of other media that on the whole do not benefit us in any way. Instead of helping us, this type of information actually serves as a distraction because it directs our attention in the wrong direction. Being exposed to too much of this kind of information can lead to developing damaging mindsets and patterns of behaviour, distancing us further from our goals and optimal existence. It can even lead to forgetting what our goals are in the first place!

Evidently, both the source and quality of information are of great importance to us. Information is so essential to our lives that it can be categorically stated that in our modern world, in the time we live in, information is everything.

To all intents and purposes, we all begin life from the same starting point. Once life begins, the race into the unknown is full of both obstacles and revelations. We are driven by the inner desire we all share – to fulfil our potential and achieve excellence. This desire has a positive effect on our development because people who do not make daily efforts to improve - to become better in some sense than they were the previous day - are missing the real point of life. Life should be understood as an opportunity to face the unknown, individually and collectively, and to advance and optimise all aspects of human existence. In the game of life some achieve a lot, but some clearly don't. People who are able to discern and assimilate the type of information that will enable them to move, improve and continue to progress a step further each day, get the fulfilment and satisfaction we all seek.

The first step in achieving personal excellence is obtaining the right information. But what is the right information? Is it the same for all of us? Is the information ultimately the answer to all our problems, questions and struggles?

Unfortunately, it is not that simple. There isn't a single source of information that would on its own enable us to achieve universal fulfilment. The only advantage of acquiring information comes from the constant interaction between experience and obtaining new knowledge, a cycle which takes us into a permanent process of self-improvement. You can never reach the final stage in perfecting yourself! Personal excellence exists for us only in the form of continuously progressing within the complex interaction of different forms of human expression.

After you have set your goals, you have to concentrate on selecting the right information to give structure to the knowledge you need for self-improvement. The only way we know that we are making correct choices when it comes to information, is through our experience. If, in reality, you are getting closer to achieving your goals, that is a clear indication that you are selecting and using the right kinds of information. If your goals seem well-chosen, but you are not getting any closer to achieving them, you are on the wrong track. In that case, you must revise your sources of information and choose something that works better.

If you have set yourself a goal of getting promoted within a year into a position of a business analyst, for instance, you must start by making efforts to obtain as much information as possible about that specific job. Speak to successful business analysts, learn from them, try to discover what they have in common, and read up on the necessary skills that will help you to succeed. Surround yourself with people who understand your desire and ambition, who are positive and supportive and make you feel good when you are in their presence. Get as much positive energy from them as you can; start breathing and feeling success. Imagine and visualise yourself as already there, a successful business analyst, and live that image as if it were actually happening. Let the properly selected information generate the knowledge necessary for achieving your goal.

You have to develop a keen sense for the right kind of information. Knowledge is the first step in the process of self-improvement, and we must not fail to acquire it through exposing ourselves to the right kind of information. Some people get it right from the start, but not many. Most of us, in fact, have to strive continually, to actively seek for as long as it takes to get to the right kind of information. Obtaining it leads to acquiring knowledge that allows us to get to the peaks we have envisaged.

Once we feel that the information we have obtained is correct and that we have a solid foundation in knowledge, we have to find motivation to put that knowledge into practice. We have to prove on a practical level that we wish to make changes towards becoming happier, more confident and productive. In our competitive living environment we want all kinds of affirmation. Our complex being can improve itself only if it is completely fulfilled. This takes us to the next stage of self-improvement: Motivation.

Motivation

We should start discussing motivation with the explanation of values, as they are among the most powerful motivational tools we have. The impact of values on creating and achieving motivation that has the power to take us from information to action, cannot be underestimated.

Our urge to find the final, universal answer to every question that matters to us is unstoppable. It derives from the instinct that makes us seek comfort and security, achieved with as little effort on our part as possible, and without delay. We always want everything for not much in return. But finding the truth often requires more than that; the truth comes to those who are ready to explore, to face their fears, to hear the unexpected, and most of all, who are ready to change.

When we start thinking about values we are at first struck by a comforting realisation: we already have a foundation, we can begin by seeking out universal values and finding the method of selecting those that are most beneficial to our development. However, absolute values that would work for all of us do not exist. Values vary from culture to culture and they are different in different times. The selection and the order of priority of values which make one culture happy and contended may not have anything beneficial to offer to another. The system of values that was widely accepted in the past, for example, would be hardly appropriate today.

In a way, we are simply a reflection of the times and the culture we live in. We cannot help being driven by great ethical ideals of our time such as democracy, tolerance, protection of the environment, equal opportunities and charity. These ideals are shaping our perception of values and playing a crucial role in their formation and assimilation. Our values are basically a reflection of our times and the culture we have inherited from generations before us.

There are several areas we should look at closely when discussing values. We build our values around health, freedom, love, relationships, work and wealth. These are the most important aspects of our lives and we generate our values in relation to them. Differences in the choice of values and in the order of priority we assign to them undoubtedly occur between individuals, as they do between different cultures. Some people move and adopt a different culture to their own in order to live by values that they feel suit them better. However, even within the same culture, different individuals make different choices, giving precedence to certain values over others. Individually, we reflect very different needs and goals, therefore our temporary values are unlikely to be the same.

We can broadly categorise values into those that are more general and those that are more specific. Values which are attainable quickly, through setting short-term goals, guide us towards more general values, which require achieving long-term goals. For example, if we pursue better health as dictated by one of our general values, eating healthily becomes a more specific value that can be achieved by setting a short-term goal, such as eating only healthy food for at least a week. The consistency in implementing such short-term goals helps us to create a good lifestyle and develop habits that will move us towards achieving harmony with our more general, fundamental values.

Achieving harmony with our fundamental values can never be an accomplished fact; it is rather a continuous process of self-improvement that lasts a lifetime. We can never reach the final stage of love; we can only love constantly, thus benefiting from deeper experiences of love over time. We cannot achieve absolute health as some irreversible state, we can only live healthily day to day, constantly improving our lifestyle and our habits, deriving pleasure from the benefits they bring throughout the process.

Values are not something that we can simply get, or buy; they are a powerful steady light that is at the end of an endless tunnel. Each time we take a step closer to the light we become more fulfilled, enriched by excellence that comes from living in harmony with our values.

Selection of values: health, freedom, love, relationships, work, money

In the process of attainment, our goals are our fuel. Setting goals and achieving them facilitates smooth progress towards our ultimate values. Once we determine which values are most important to us we have to develop a strategy to enable us to uphold them. This can only happen through regularly setting ourselves tasks and striving towards them – a process known as goal-setting. Without clear goals we are unable to improve because we lack direction. Our goals map out our paths to excellence.

We can talk about short, medium and long-term goals. Short-term goals are best used as first steps, the goals we feel we can achieve in a short time. Setting ourselves short-term goals builds our confidence and motivates us to go on to higher achievements. For example, if your long-term goal is to get a degree in science which takes four years of study, your short-term goal would be to grasp a certain amount of material each week. If you fulfil that goal week after week, you will inevitably start to feel confident about achieving your long-term goal, a degree, and this confidence will further motivate you to continue your studies.

A medium-term goal might be to successfully complete the first year of study, passing all the required exams with good marks. Achieving a medium-term goal gives you still more confidence and motivation. Once you achieve a particular medium-term goal you have to revert back to setting the short-term goals for the following stage. The success of regularly fulfilling smaller, easier tasks can only encourage you to use the same technique to achieve your next medium-term goal, such as successfully finishing the second year of study.

Consistency in goal-setting and achieving your short and medium-term goals ultimately leads to achieving your designated long term-goal, such as a degree in science. The long-term goal provided direction and focus for the entire process,.

Different fundamental values obviously require us to set goals in different areas, such as health, relationships, work, and spiritual life. You can have different goals set out in front of you, but as long as they are properly selected and set, and you are persistent in achieving them, you will be living successfully. Results that come from achieving short, medium and long-term goals are the best and only proof that you are living according to your fundamental values

If you select wisely which values to endorse and start working towards them through setting targets and goals, you acquire everything that is necessary for a person to become motivated. The fundamental purpose of life reveals itself, leaving you with no other option but to act! Once discovered, the meaning of existence is an extremely powerful notion, capable of charging our mental forces to accomplish an action.

There are many reasons why people find it difficult to build up sufficient motivation to make the change and improve themselves. By constantly optimising our mental and physical capabilities, we create a better relationship with ourselves and with others; we are receiving more and giving more. Some of the reasons for loosing motivation are: fear of the unknown, fear of challenge, fear of rejection, fear of failure, living to please others, reacting instead of creating and lacking vision. Let's take a look at a couple of ideas that can help self-motivation.

Many people live in the past. They constantly think about things that happened, or could have happened in the past. Past outcomes become excuses in the present; they are typically the reason people give for backing away from doing something new, something that might challenge them. The past often creates feelings of guilt, and guilt simply kills creativity and motivation. On the other hand, there are people who constantly project into the future. Their dreams and imaginations become their reality; they dwell on them too much and this ruins the present for them. Constantly dwelling on what might happen in the future, imagining and visualising it, inevitably provokes fear that we will not be able to achieve the mental picture we have created, and this is again detrimental to our lives in the present. Dreams and aspirations can become a strong point of motivation only if you decide to live in the present! You can achieve happiness, satisfaction and fulfilment only by living now, in this very moment, by learning and persistently acting on that knowledge.

If you decide to live your life as it is, without changing anything, without challenging yourself with new experiences and new situations, you will always live the same life. Nothing will get better and your physical and mental abilities will stagnate, until they start diminishing with age. If you are happy with that, fine. But if you want more from life you have to change both your behaviour and your strategy. If something is unfamiliar, face it. The only way to discover it is to plunge head-first into it. If you fear a certain challenge, do it! The only way to beat fear is to face it. The feeling you experience after overcoming fear and moving another step forward will provide you with sufficient motivation and energy to continue on the road to self-excellence.

If you don't want to be one of those people who always complain about being bored and leading an unfulfilling life, then don't live the same day twice! Every day should be taken as an opportunity to face new experiences, new challenges, and reveal the new you. You cannot live exclusively within your comfort zone, backing away from new experiences and criticising everything that is different from your current situation. You have to leave your comfort zone and face the challenge of improvement, the wonderful challenge that leads you to freedom. Hold your head up and sail towards the better you.

People around you play a very important role in the process of motivation and self-improvement. We are social beings. We need social interaction in order to understand who we are, and to understand others. The need to interact, to communicate, is a fundamental factor in our mental and physical development. But is our social milieu necessarily supportive of our efforts to improve, to live better? Not always. Some people in your circle will be negative and jealous and become fearful as you improve. The change in you will remind them of their own apathy and inertia. Such friends will only pull you back into the old you. If you examine the goals you have abandoned and realise that people from your surroundings had explicitly or implicitly influenced you to give up, this means that you have to start choosing people around you more cautiously. You have to become more circumspect in selecting people you can trust, and seek out those with whom you want to share your successes and new experiences. Choose to spend time with positive people, try to find friends who are supportive, excited and happy about your achievements. They will also benefit from being around you; you may inspire them to try to improve themselves. The right social environment is extremely important for both motivation and inspiration.

Many people live their lives entirely according to the expectations of others. We can never free ourselves from the expectations of others, and at certain stages of life we all live by them – as young children, for example, when we live almost entirely according to the expectations of our parents. However, instead of this being just a phase, many of us remain locked forever in that situation of living life to please others. If we are constantly thinking about how others will react to the decisions we make we forget our own ideas, thoughts and future plans. We must live our own lives, and live them in the present moment, because that is the only time we have. Let others learn about you and judge you by your behaviour, let them appreciate and respect who you really are. Find your own way of making that change and take charge of your life.

In the process of self-motivation, knowing your inner self is immensely important. Learning about oneself is probably the greatest task that a person can aspire to. Everything we want to know about ourselves will be revealed in the course of a lifetime, but we have to persist in making efforts, because only through constantly changing and developing do we keep discovering new things about ourselves

Start with discovering yourself now. Look inside and try to find what it is that makes you happy, satisfied and hungry for success. Seek out your fears and find out what makes you upset and angry. Understand what challenges you intellectually, discover the arts that feed your soul, and find what you have to offer to others. You have to learn what it is that you really want. Once you know what it is you can focus on it, setting your goals accordingly and fuelling your motivation to actually achieve it.

At the same time, you have to know what you want from life. You cannot copy others in their pursuit of excellence. What other people want has nothing to do with you.

Strong willpower is your best tool for conquering yourself. We all have it, but not all of us develop and use it to the same extent. Developing willpower is the fastest technique for realising your goals and living in accordance with your fundamental values. Create the vision which will give you the reason to take action and to make things happen. Create your own mental picture of worthiness and success.

You will discover a great sense of personal fulfilment in the continuous process of optimising your inner powers.

Action

Welcome to the real world! Welcome to life on a practical level, where one word means literally everything: action. Our interactions, our movements, all of our achievements are nothing but action – information applied in a practical sense. We need action to materialise our ideas. The force that connects information and action is motivation. This is the process in which information, supported by motivation, evolves into action.

There is an old saying that actions speak louder than any combination of words. At the same time, action can be seen as a sign of the aptness of one's approach. Action is the final stage in the natural order of events: desire, information, motivation and action. Without action, the desired process of achievement will never reach the stage of practical application. Progress and improvement will be buried and lost in the realm of theoretical and contemplative intellectual experiment.

- Without action there is no change.
- Without action there is no improvement.
- Consistency in life stops with the lack of action.
- We can also understand action as an aspect of energy and a supreme purpose in life.

Quite often people uncover information which is vital for their personal improvement and they even get motivated to act on that information, but they never make the necessary steps towards real action. Great ideas remain no more than ideas, potentials waiting to be realised. But if they are not materialised, over time even the clearest ideas deteriorate and fade away. There are many reasons why some people never take the final step, why they never embark upon action, even when they know it is the only way to improve themselves further. The most common reasons for the lack of action are:

- Weak desire
- Hesitation
- Fear of failure
- Fear of change
- Fear of hard work

If your desire for improvement is not strong enough from the very beginning, action will never happen. Regardless of the information and motivation that you may have, the desire to move forward must be strong enough to bring about action. Desires can be different, as our expectations and needs are different, resulting in different achievements. But regardless of which course of action you take, your desire has to be strong enough to incite action.

Hesitation is another reason that can prevent action from happening. Weak desire creates a perfect breeding ground for hesitation.

Hesitation emerges as a result of an unclear mental picture of what it is you need and how much you really want it. Low self-confidence, which results from a lack of information and motivation, can also provoke hesitation. The best antidote to hesitation is a stronger sense of desire, along with access to relevant information and a higher level of motivation. Once you have armed yourself with these powerful mental tools, there should be no room for hesitation, and action should arise naturally.

A fear of failure is yet another reason why sometimes we are unable to act. People do not want to imagine failing to accomplish a task. For some, failure is simply too frightening and it effectively stops them from initiating the chain of events necessary to bring about action. Still, a strong desire, adequate knowledge and strong motivation are all you need to overcome the fear of failure. In the face of failure you have to be ready to try again, with a renewed enthusiasm and confidence until you succeed at making the change. Consistency in approach will award you with success. Many great discoveries in history were made only after centuries of blunders and failed attempts. But humanity's strong desire, high motivation and understanding of the value of consistency meant that failures did not ultimately deter us. They were simply obstacles that had to be eliminated. Every failure you suffer along the way should be viewed as a valuable experience that has the power to make you stronger, more decisive and more determined to accomplish your goal. The more you struggle on the road to achievement, the more you will appreciate the journey and enjoy the results that come from overcoming obstacles along the way. Fear of change is a common stumbling block that can hinder our ability to act. Living exclusively within a comfort zone you get used to the security of your 'soul cage', it inspires confidence that feels like freedom. But being imprisoned inside this cage, where everything is placid and nothing is provoking, disturbing or exciting, creates a life in which nothing more can happen. Even when you generate a drop of aspiration to leave the confines of your cage to try something new, even if you acquire the correct information and the motivation to act, the fear of change may still be stronger and prevent you from acting. Common questions that arise when you contemplate taking action towards change are:

- Am I going to like the new me?
- Am I going to be accepted when I change?
- Can I be happy outside my comfort zone?
- Will the change bring more responsibilities?
- Is change simply going to lead me into another cage?
- Will the new me be about me only, or will I have to help others as well?

Change should always be seen as a single stage in continuous improvement, a stepping-stone towards the better and stronger you. Someone that you like, someone who is ready to exchange new information and experiences with others.

Fear of hard work is another frequent obstacle that gets in the way of creative action. Hard work is seen as something that takes us away from our happiness and disturbs the tranquillity of our every-day life. But, faced with a choice between relatively easy work that leads to mediocrity, or harder work that leads to a more proactive life which is full of opportunities, we would do well to favour the latter. Rather than being a hindrance, adopting hard work as second nature, something that we accept as useful and commendable, will serve us well in our battle to better ourselves.

It is not hard work that deters people from action, it is their approach to hard work and their understanding of it. If we do not even begin something because it seems like hard work, the problem lies in the fact that we have never actually attempted it. Things that we have done in the past are never a problem – only things that we have never done before can cause confusion and fear. We have all done things in the past we can call hard work. If you look at it closely you realise that hard work only helped you to get where you are now. All we need to do in order to progress is remind ourselves of past situations when hard work produced great results. To repeat the same success, we have to embrace hard work and new challenges with enthusiasm. Choosing to work hard has to be understood as a freedom and a privilege of human existence, because it represents our own decision to engage all of our mental and physical forces in order to progress.

Physical Activity through Exercise

Through the process of evolution human species developed unique physical characteristics. What makes us most obviously different from other closely related species is our distinctive erect posture. Our upright bodies allow us to perform certain physical activities far more efficiently and safely than other species. Our anatomy and physiology give the best clues for identifying the safest and most productive physical activities for the human body.

In the context of deciding on the best sporting activity available to us today we are frequently baffled by exposure to incompetent sources of information. If we are searching for the type of exercise that will make us fitter, stronger, and more resistant to illness, we must first learn what it means to be fit. Secondly, we must learn what strength is and how to increase it. Thirdly, we must become aware of the fact that the immune system responds directly and positively to a stronger and more robust physique.

Today we are witnessing a dramatic increase in orthopaedic injuries caused by activities that involve running. Injuries of the foot, ankle, Achilles tendon, knee, hip joint, lower and upper back and other areas, represent an every-day reality for both recreational and professional runners. In addition, runners have to deal with a diminished hormonal response and endocrine reaction, and an overall weakening in bone density. Despite this, people still believe that any form of running is the best possible choice of physical activity for human fitness. However, as I am about to show you, the popularity of so-called aerobic activities is based upon two major factors: a lack of information and the desire for comfort.

We first have to understand that humans, being erect mammals, are not built for running. It is the least natural activity for us and the main reason why running is so detrimental to our bodies. Our spine, limbs, joints, and indeed complete biomechanics are designed for walking and performing other, much safer physical activities. It was sudden bursts of explosive movement, with a completely different combination of muscle groups to those required for slow, low-intensity, long-duration aerobic activities, that were responsible for our survival. The skills that allowed us to survive for so long did not include the ability to jog comfortably for hours or to perform step aerobics. Our survival skills required sprinting, heavy lifting, throwing, wrestling, fighting, and killing! Humans survived due to extremely intense and complex muscular activity that allowed us to be permanently ready for the unexpected in our harsh and merciless environment. The key to understanding this is to take a look at our heavily built skeleton – our big joints and exceedingly strong connective tissues. These, along with the ability to instantly respond hormonally and to be ready at a moment's notice to strike back with full force, have proved indispensible for our survival. It is a fact that the dominant muscle fibre in the human body is the fast-twitch, white muscle fibre, which is optimised for short-duration, high-intensity activity. Genetically, we are built better for hard, intense exertion than for slow, low-intensity, long-duration activity.

Hormonally as well, we respond better to high-intensity activities, which are known to increase the production of crucial hormones – growth hormone and testosterone. These hormones are responsible for our growth, strength, fertility, sufficient bone density, strong immunity, a healthy cardiovascular system, higher red blood cells count and an efficient reproductive system. At the other end of the spectrum of physical activities, long-duration, low-intensity activities such as running actually decrease the production of these essential hormones.

We can summarise that, when it comes to human physical activity, a major division is between:

1) low-intensity, long-duration activities
   and
2) high-intensity, short-duration activities

The obvious difference between these two activities is in the intensity with which they are performed. Low-intensity activities allow a long period of non-stop engagement. Jogging, cycling, swimming, aerobics and other similar activities engage only some of the body systems and only up to a certain level. People spend hours doing them and this makes them feel like they have achieved something, but the overall impact on their body can never be high enough to trigger an optimal response.

When we talk about lifestyle change and overcoming the increasing levels of work-related stress while at the same time making further progress, we have to look at the optimal performance of all of our body systems. We need to consider the effects of increased metabolism and insulin sensitivity, fat loss, stronger muscles, healthier and stronger bones, joints and connective tissues. We must think about the benefits of a strong cardiovascular system, efficient endocrine system, better digestion, detoxification, better sleep, more self-confidence and better motivation and creativity.

To make these kinds of changes we require a particular type of physical activity. We need a higher impact and a stronger stimulus that will trigger the body into a positive response. What we desperately need is a high-intensity physical activity. We need high intensity resistance training!

Nutrition through Healthy Eating

There is a lot of information available on the subject of healthy eating and the right choice of food. Almost everyone knows or believes that they know what constitutes a healthy diet and which foods should be avoided. We live in an age in which people believe they know more about healthy nutrition than ever before, yet this results in entirely unexpected and unwelcome outcomes.

We have never been exposed to more information about healthy diet and we have never been more attentive to it than we are today. Take, for example, the hype about fat. Never in our history have we had such a wide choice of low-fat products as we have today; almost everything on the shelves in our supermarkets is low-fat. This is because the medical establishment, with generous assistance from all forms of media, has made people scared to death of fat! And yet, at a time before the Second World War, when there where no low-fat products to buy, the levels of cardiovascular disease, cancer, diabetes and obesity were much lower. In modern times it would appear that knowledge and experience serve more as a detriment than an advantage. Throughout our evolution, up to the time of agrarian reform which slowly set us on the course of becoming omnivores, we were primarily meat-eaters and our food consisted of much more fat than it does today. And yet in those times people did not suffer from the chronic diseases that we suffer from today! It is a paradox that more 'knowledge' and information about food seems to have resulted in an unprecedented increase in the incidence of illness and death.

Our physiology (our digestion, metabolism, hormonal and cardiovascular systems) has developed over time. We did not make conscious decisions about things like our biochemistry, anatomy, optimal joint rotation or the perfect balance of our bodily systems. All our bodily systems and their functions are the product of our ability to adapt to a living environment and function efficiently within it, and ultimately, to survive. Our living environment and the types of food it offered, which nourished and allowed us to survive as a species, have dictated the direction in which we have adapted to become what we are today.

According to some scientists, we emerged into our present form some 150.000 years ago! We may have come a long way since then, but the food that was available to us has become a part our biochemical composition. Our physiology today is simply the result of the best response to the immediate living environment we could produce over some 140.000 years. That was a sufficient amount of time to allow changes in our genetic structure so that we could adapt and improve in response to the natural world around us. Our ability to digest meat, vegetables and fruit with maximum efficiency was reflected in our superior health, vigour, strength and a minimum risk of developing chronic diseases as we know them today. Our inability to cope with diets lacking in protein, fibre, minerals, vitamins and water has resulted in a number of chronic diseases that are currently devastating our civilisation. We have never adjusted to consuming foods that are low in protein, water and fibre, while at the same time extremely dense in starchy carbohydrates, hydrogenated fats and the combination of polyunsaturated fats.

We were first introduced to starch from grains, and not long after, the human race was exposed to the biggest edible killer of them all – refined sugar. Starch and refined sugar have reduced the length and quality of life more than any other factor in our living environment in last 10.000 years. The percentage of carbohydrates found in natural foods ranges from 3% in vegetables to no more than 13% in fruits. Therefore, if we followed a diet recommended by nature, with the right percentage of natural sugar and containing lots of fibre and water, it would be impossible to consume too many carbohydrates. It would take six to seven apples or three kilograms of tomatoes to match the amount of carbohydrates found in a typical meal with pasta, rice or mashed potatoes!

For most of our evolution, the nature and composition of fats in our diet was such that our physiology adapted and responded perfectly to what we ate. Monounsaturated fats were abundant in foods such as nuts and vegetables, while polyunsaturated fats were found in the right balance and quantity in the meat of wild animals and fish. With the introduction of grains into our diet (after the discovery of agriculture) the daily consumption of meat, fruits and vegetables dropped dramatically, effectively decreasing the amount and combination of healthy fats in our diet. Since domesticated animals have also been introduced to grains, the composition of their meat has also changed. The amount and types of fat in their meat is now completely different to that found in the meat of wild animals, which fed on wild foods rather than on cultivated grains. From whichever angle we look at our diet, we have to acknowledge that we are not eating the types of food that would be the most conducive to our development. Our diet is predominantly composed of grains and grain products, and this results in an extremely high carbohydrate intake which causes a range of chronic diseases frequently seen today. The types and the amount of fat we consume today from meat and different kinds of oil are causing health problems which were unknown to humanity for the most part of our evolution, when our diet was governed by nature.

Now lets take a look at enzymes. Have you ever heard of enzymes? They are the most powerful and influential chemicals found in fresh foods, but food manufacturers and nutritionists rarely mention them. Instead, in their efforts to win the hearts and minds of consumers, we are bombarded with information about the amount of fat or sugar in our food and suggestions of what constitutes 'healthy' daily amounts. You never hear a word about enzymes; the average person's immediate reaction when they are mentioned is to think about washing powder! The fact is, enzymes are very efficient catalysts for biochemical reactions and, as a component of natural fresh foods, have a tremendously beneficial effect on our health. The problem is that they are active only in fresh foods and are actually eliminated from the same foods once they are frozen, dried or cooked. How often do you eat fresh fruit and salads – daily, weekly, monthly? This is essentially how often you supply these powerful enzymes to your body. Every meal you have during the day should consist of 2/3 of fruit and vegetables and 1/3 of lean meats.

Nature has created us and nature will eliminate us if we stop following the fundamental principles upon which we have evolved. Compared to the diet of our ancestors, the selection, amount, composition and quality of food we eat today has completely changed. The amount of protein has dramatically decreased while the amount of carbohydrates has dramatically increased. The fats we consume today with such devastating effects on our health were not available to our ancestors. At the same time, there isn't a modern diet that can match the amount of properly balanced healthy fats that our ancestors consumed. The amount of potassium we get from our food has decreased while the amount of sodium has increased enormously! Today we also eat much less fibre than our ancestors, while the amount of essential minerals and vitamins has been almost halved compared to our diet of some 10.000 years ago.

So, how do these discrepancies in or current dietary habits affect our health? If we were not designed to consume the food that we are consuming today globally in huge amounts and we have not adapted to it over time, how do we cope? Not surprisingly, the health statistics are devastating. These days we suffer from illnesses that have never been as prevalent before: obesity, diabetes, cancer, cardiovascular disease, allergies, tooth decay, bone deformities, and other illnesses which were unknown to our ancestors on the scale and magnitude that we know them today.

Obviously, something is very wrong. Despite frantic attempts by governments to deal with the consequences of poor nutrition by pumping vast amounts of money into educating the general public, promoting 'healthy eating' in the media and banning advertising of unhealthy foods, imposing limits on the amount of salt and sugar, banning vending machines in schools and many other quick-fix measures, the results are still less than encouraging. Obesity is generally on the rise, with children being affected more than ever before. Diabetes in children has also reached alarming proportions, while the incidence of diabetes 2 is higher than ever in the general population. Cardiovascular disease continues to be the leading cause of death in adults. These facts point to one of two conclusions: either our knowledge about food and diet is wrong, or it is not being applied properly. Knowing the solution is one thing, but using that knowledge to act and change our situation is something completely different.

To summarise, we live in an age when we think we know everything there is to know about food, but despite this, we are not experiencing a great deal of progress in our overall health. This is the case primarily because of the following reasons:

- Our knowledge about food and diet is generally wrong.
- Where poor results were obtained by applying this 'knowledge', not much corrective action has been taken.
- Our dogmatic approach to things leads to denial of any misreading of the situation on our part.
- Our fear of change and the need to maintain the status quo.
- Our unwillingness to question the official trends and thinking in nutritional science and theory.

Let us start with the first point: that our knowledge about healthy eating is incorrect. In our society today, to disagree with something that has been established as 'official' for more than six decades is considered a form of heresy. Once a piece of information is 'established' as scientific fact and we start to follow it as though it were a religious belief, questioning or interfering with it in any way becomes extremely difficult. On the other hand, telling people that everything they know about feeding themselves and their children is wrong and should be changed, is not easy either. Even when faced with hard evidence from ailments such as tooth decay, obesity, heart disease, diabetes and a general decline in overall health, people would still rather stick to their old beliefs than consider new ones. The idea of change, of entering the unknown, often seems too threatening. Living in our comfort zone is far more attractive than attempting to wrestle with the causes of the loss of so many lives per year. Comfort and selfishness indeed go hand in hand.

Now let's take a look at the second point: despite copious government advice about healthy eating habits, our general health is deteriorating and nobody (including fitness specialists, the general public, medical personnel and nutritional bodies) has ever attempted to question the accuracy of this information. We are silent witnesses to a steady increase in obesity, diabetes, and heart disease, and we still live under the illusion that these conditions happen only to other people and will never happen to us. If the current situation with health and nutrition information and advice continues, soon every one of us will have the 'privilege' of developing one or another form of self-inflicted chronic disease!

When it comes to our dogmatic reluctance to address any of our own misconceptions, we still attach too much importance to various dietary theories, while not displaying enough courage and depth of understanding to enable us to rectify ideas that may be flawed. If something doesn't produce positive results we have to be ready and willing to face it, challenge it and change it. If a scientific theory comes up with unsatisfactory results, we have to challenge that theoretical approach and change it. Ultimately, what counts is a positive result, which, in the context of our discussion, is represented by good health for every individual and for the human race as a whole. If we are not managing to get positive results, everything offered to us in the form of science, religion and philosophy has to be revised time and again, for as long as it takes, until we start achieving success. As humans strive towards the truth, there can be no room for dogmatic, unproductive stubbornness.

It is a common practice among nutritionists to simply provide reassurance and gratification to individuals who suffer from diet-related illnesses without explaining the fundamentals of human physiology and how it responds to food. In addition, once the right information is conveyed and understood, we have to find the motivation and initiate action in order to resolve existing problems. Our over-emphasis on mental and emotional states above our physical existence has brought us to the point we are at now. We now feel more secure mentally and emotionally, mostly due to our incorrect eating habits and our ignorance of physical fitness, and this is more true now than ever before! It is crucial that we begin to understand that without physical existence, no other existence is possible, and that because of this our body has to become our temple again, providing us with everything that makes us human. If our physical existence is compromised, everything else that comes out of it suffers accordingly. Health and physical fitness should be reintroduced to us through proper education and the implementation of healthy lifestyle methods that will bring and maintain positive results. In many ways it seems that we have reached the point of no return. However, we may still have a chance of turning things around by going back to the original human diet that has for millions of years granted us

strength, vitality, strong immunity and an absence of self-inflicted chronic diseases.

If religion has been criticised for its rigid, dogmatic approach
that doesn't allow any compromise or challenge, then the same
can be said of science. It usually takes decades to refute even
the smallest part of a scientifically accepted system, regardless
of the type of science. No matter what science throws up, in this
case the science of nutrition, we rarely challenge or question it.
We just shuffle scientific dogmas around in order to try to prove
them right in practice. If the price we pay for this is millions of
destroyed lives around the world, that may be fatal for the human
race, but not for the science of nutrition as it is currently viewed.

Many factors influence what is going to be labelled as scientific
research or scientific discovery. The most powerful of these
factors is undoubtedly 'political correctness', but there are also
commercial forces at work. Universities, for example, are paid
large amounts of money to support existing theories that enable corporations to make enormous profits. The grain industry,
which has enormous financial resources, will always support
theories which demonstrate the health benefits of the high consumption of grain in our daily diet. Similarly, petroleum industry will support scientists whose findings sustain the notion that
we need petroleum-based sources of energy in order to maintain
high standards of living in the developed world. The same is
true of every industry that uses its financial clout to influence

science. The real problems that an ordinary person faces today are directly related to the detrimental side effects of our 'healthy' eating habits which are supported by experts, the medical establishment and accountable government bodies. In the face of all this, we are still reluctant to question the current dogmas in the field of nutrition. We continue making whole-grain sandwiches full of butter and cheese without regard to the likelihood of developing high blood pressure or insulin resistance from this supposedly healthy food.

Food

A few things about food need to be considered again because its perception and significance have been greatly misunderstood over the last sixty years.

First of all, we know that in order to live, we have to eat. We can therefore agree that we eat to live. It is very important for people living in this current era to make this crucial 'discovery'.

As physical entities, we can only exist and function if we provide a steady stream of nutrients to our system. Our vital tissues are composed of macronutrients such as proteins, fats and carbohydrates. Skin, muscles, hair, nails, heart, liver, lungs, blood, are all made of macronutrients. We can get these essential components only from the food that we eat. We are entirely dependent on food and have to eat the necessary amounts of certain types of food, several times a day, every day.

Since the time of the ancient Greeks and their efforts to understand human nature, mind, body and spirit, one macronutrient in particular has triggered the attention of the wise and earned itself a special name: protein. The name derives from the Greek word *proteios*, which means 'primary, first'. So, as far as 2.300 years ago, proteios was known to be the most important macronutrient in the human body, a building block to all our tissues including muscles, skin, bones, internal organs, hair, nails and blood cells. We call it protein today, but we use the name without truly understanding the meaning of the word, which renders us incapable of deciphering the message contained within it which passed down through the ages. In modern times, the most important component of our daily food intake has been assigned the least priority. Protein cannot compete with 'tasty' fat and sugar in our daily diet. Along with salt, fat and complex carbohydrates will always triumph in the war against protein. If we add to the equation the high cost of good-quality food which is rich in protein, it becomes clear which of these macronutrients is likely to be the winner.

The fact is that food is heavily politicised today. Large food corporations are engaged in constant competition with each other; they act mercilessly and with a warped sense of right and wrong. They are not interested in the lasting consequences that their products have on the consumer. They seek only one thing: profit. They have introduced every ingredient they can think of into food to create addiction and make consumers dependent on their products. The most powerful of these is the addiction to sugar, or more precisely, the addiction to all types of carbohydrates.

By simply introducing carbohydrates into our food, food manufacturers render it highly addictive to anyone who consumes it. This is because of the way our hormonal system responds to the food that we eat. A high intake of all types of carbohydrates causes over-production of insulin. By eating cereals, bread, rice, pasta, cakes, and other foods that are dense in carbohydrates, we increase the blood-sugar levels well above the normal. High levels of blood-sugar compel the body to produce insulin in order to bring them down. The problem is that a high intake of carbohydrates forces the production of extremely high levels of insulin. Such high levels of insulin do not only lower the blood sugar to a normal level, but they lower it to well below normal levels! In such circumstances, by eating carbohydrates, a person actually ends up with very low blood sugar, which manifests itself in various negative ways such as tiredness, exhaustion, lethargy, nervousness and hunger. The hunger caused by a sudden drop in sugar levels is basically a carbohydrate craving. And the easiest way to fix the problem, even if only temporarily, is to ingest some more carbohydrates!

Once your system is overloaded with carbohydrates again, the exact same insulin reaction will follow and you will end up resorting to quick fixes throughout the day and consuming carbohydrates again and again to alleviate the situation. It is quite common for people to consume as many as 10 carbohydrate-rich servings of food each day to feed such addictions! In cases like these the body becomes flooded with insulin and we enter what can be called a 'vicious insulin cycle'. As long as we rely on carbohydrates as the only energy source worth considering, over-production of insulin and its consequences will be a daily reality for us.

The most obvious side-effect of insulin hyper-production is obesity, but there are also lesser known links with diabetes, hypertension, high cholesterol levels, high risk of strokes and hormonal imbalance. The only solution to these problems would be to switch to another energy source altogether – our very own body fat!

Our obsession with calories, the fanaticism with which we check recommended daily calorie requirements and whether we are eating too many or too few per day, shows how easily a marginal threat can grab all the attention. Food carries calories, but regulating the amount of calories that we consume on a daily basis should be performed as an instinctive physiological response rather than a dogmatic mathematical formula. The problem is that we do not have a recognisable physiological response that would deter us from eating certain foods or certain amount of food in a single sitting. Today, we have to be told what type, amount and composition of food is beneficial to us. Soon we are going to be told how to breathe! Our instinctive knowledge of what constitutes good food for us and its proper amounts has been replaced by the suggestions of 'experts', the art of cooking, social preferences for certain types of food, super snacks, etc.

The food industry today has been reduced to a craft of finding new substances that the human body can absorb without immediate side-effects, making them tasty by filling them with salt and sugar, and packing them into bright, colourful packaging. Moreover, we are experiencing the need for ongoing research into how much food the human body can absorb and how much the human gut can stretch. How long does the pancreas continue producing insulin if it is bombarded by carbohydrates from early on in life, and how much body weight can an individual sustain? We know only too well the effects of such dangerous conditions and symptoms: chronic disease, obesity, tooth decay, loss of mobility, premature aging and early death.

So, do we have anything to guide us to acquiring and maintaining healthy and sensible eating habits? How can we recognise the right foods and identify the right quantities?

We did not have cookbooks, low-fat products, government guidelines or celebrities promoting the latest super cereals while we were developing as a species. We ate only food that had been consumed by humans for millions of years – food that was created for us and that did not cause chronic diseases that plague modern civilisation. Our ancestors were not affected by obesity, diabetes, or hypertension. These common killers of today were completely unknown to them. They did not have toothpaste, dentists or super supplements to keep them healthy!

If we compare ourselves to our ancestors, what emerges is a grim picture of a race afflicted by weak health and physical disadvantages, heavily dependent on medication and addicted to all the wrong foods and chemicals.

So, how did we manage to survive without technology and drugs, and to filter and pass on superior genetic material to new generations? What did we eat, and how did we know what not to eat and how to control our appetite?

Foods that have been consumed for millions of years had an effect on the development of our digestive and other bodily systems. Our food was mainly composed of water, fibre, protein, fat and a few carbohydrates. It was very rich in essential minerals and vitamins which play important role in the process of digestion and absorption, blood formation, bone metabolism and muscle contraction among others. The basic human diet consisted, as it still does, of meat, fruit and vegetables. The proportion of macronutrients, water and fibre, in this diet provides us with the perfect balance of protein, fat, carbohydrate, water and fibre, which enables us to live long and healthy lives.

Our bodies are built to take care of themselves. We always recognise when to stop when we are eating natural, healthy food, which is normally bulky but relatively low in calories. Besides, food that is mainly composed of water and fibre cannot carry too many calories anyway. It is our modern food such as biscuits, cakes, sweets, bread, rice, cereals and chips, which are dry and full of sugar and fat, that can overload the system with calories. At the same time, although the caloric value of such food is high, these calories are 'empty' in a sense that they do not carry any valuable proteins, fats, vitamins or minerals. Once ingested, this useless food composed of empty calories can only be stored as body fat! To make things worse, in order to be metabolised, such food drains the body of essential vitamins and minerals. Natural food does not do that. As opposed to the empty food, natural food carries vitamins and minerals, easing the process of digestion and absorption and enriching other metabolic processes and tissues.

So this is the starting point of the 'science' of controlling, counting, balancing, and choosing calories. If modern food is our main choice and natural food composes only a fraction of our daily menu, then the 'science' of calories is only a mechanism to persuade people that eating modern types of food can produce fitness and vigour. The problem is that with modern diets, you have to restrict the amount of calories so much that the daily amount of calorically dense food shrinks dramatically, leaving you in despair. In this situation, it is a matter of days rather than weeks before a person slips back into consuming even more calories in order to maintain a permanent blood-sugar level. Low-calorie diets do not produce lasting results, they never did and they never will. Everyone who has tried it knows from their own experience – you can't fake it with fake food!

Eating natural food, you will never need to control calories, because you will never experience problems such as extra weight, low energy, tiredness, low blood-sugar level or hypertension. It is simply impossible to eat too much meat, fish, vegetables and fruit! We can easily regulate the daily intake of these foods. On the other hand, we cannot regulate the amount of fake food we ingest, simply because this kind of food did not exist in our evolution for long enough to create the necessary changes in our genetic makeup to allow us to adapt to it. We cannot say that we have adapted to sugary and starchy foods (according to modern science, it takes a minimum of 50.000 years of exposure to a new environmental factor to create a slight change in our genetic makeup as a response to the new living condition). Agriculture started only 10.000 years ago, so if we are waiting for evolution to help us out when it comes to sugar and fats in our diet, we have a very long time to wait.

There is another issue regarding the role of food in our lives today that needs to be addressed. As we have said, we have to eat to live. But today, a large number of people use food as a form of relief from daily stress and depression. They eat for comfort, as a reward for anything and everything. Food has become, in a way, a major obsession for modern man.

We don't eat to live anymore, we live to eat! An 'eat to live' approach is not enough any longer. If it were, we would eat much less, and less frequently. If we truly nourished ourselves in order to live better, to live longer and healthier lives, then the selection and condition of our food would change – we would eat less and stop eating refined foods containing sugar which are dense in carbohydrates and high in added fats. Simply stated, we would have to switch to food that had been created for us in the first place:

meat, fruit and vegetables. Our obsession with food would have to be replaced with the understanding of food as a necessity. We would have to learn to enjoy the taste of apples and pears, peppers and tomatoes again and forget about biscuits and chocolate!

For some, this may prove too difficult, but it is dictated by who we are, our innermost nature. These are the fuels that can enable us to maximise our intellectual and physical potential. By sticking to our own foods, our own fuels, we enable our immune system to protect us perfectly. Our energies are sapped by fighting chronic diseases, digesting almost indigestible foods, detoxifying the system, etc. If we eat a diet provided by nature, we can avoid chronic diseases and have more energy to lead creative and productive lives.

Physical Activity

Our anatomy and physiology determine the kinds of physical activity that we are capable of taking on. We walk at a certain speed but not faster, we run as far as we can, but no further. We lift heavy objects up to a certain weight but not heavier, we throw stones and javelins to a certain distance but not further; we can jump, swim, wrestle, kick and punch, but always within our own human limitations. Everything that is physically possible for us is determined by our anatomy. The length of bones in our arm determines how far we can extend while delivering a punch or throwing a stone. The length of the bones in our legs determines how fast we can run, the size of our joints such as wrists and knees determines how much weight we can lift. The size and density of our muscles determines our speed and strength, the efficiency of our metabolism determines the intensity and duration we can achieve while undertaking physical work, and a strong heart allows us to exercise with high intensity.

Human beings are capable of performing a vast range of physical activities. We take this fact for granted and rarely ask ourselves why we have such a wide range of physical ability. The answer to this question is provided by looking at our evolution. The living environment that we have been exposed to for millions of years has influenced our anatomical and physiological development.

For example, the shoulder joint's ability to rotate in different directions is a result of our constant need to use the arm to perform actions such as lifting, throwing, pushing, pulling and fighting. Only a flexible shoulder joint could have allowed such a wide variety of arm movements as was necessary for our survival.

Another example of evolutionary adaptation is the Achilles tendon. The strongest single tendon in our body, it is capable of supporting our entire weight during an intense physical activity such as sprinting, or any other explosive activity which involves the whole body. Without such a super strong tendon, we would not have been able to hunt, fight, carry heavy objects or simply run for our lives. It is true that we do not rely on these activities so much any more, but it is also true that a strong Achilles tendon played its part in enabling us to survive at all in the first place!

Everything that we are capable of performing physically today is a result of our lifestyle requirements during the course of our evolution. In order to survive, we adapted and evolved into our current form, which includes a very complex skeletal system with over 600 muscles supporting and moving that skeleton, as well as an amazing synergy of bodily systems that support each other. All this enables us to achieve a high quality of life during a span that can extend some 120 years. It is our biochemistry that makes everything function with perfection. If we accept this, what should we do to allow our body and all its systems to function perfectly, giving us health and a long life in return?

Our ancestors lived their lives the way they had to. They must have gone through a great deal of struggle and hardship and their fight to survive must have seemed impossible at times. But, by engaging their physical and intellectual abilities to the maximum, they have managed to carry on and provide us with the opportunity to continue what they have started. We have a perfect genetic potential to manage our survival and continue to improve as a species.

But, is our lifestyle today similar to the lifestyle of our ancestral Homo sapiens, who lived some 50.000 years ago? There is not much difference between us anatomically or physiologically. The only difference is that we are more vulnerable to countless diseases than they were. They did not suffer from chronic diseases that are killing modern humanity by the millions around the world. They were generally healthier than we are.

Industrial and technological progress is helping us to improve our living conditions, but at the same time it is changing our lifestyle and making us more passive, more inactive, weaker and sicker. Today everything is done with the press of a button, we use vehicles to get ourselves to a nearby shop and the machines are doing all the heavy work – we hardly ever need to make an effort any more. Physical exertion is not necessarily a part of our every-day lives; we can do everything we must do in life without even breaking into a sweat. The fact is, we do not engage physically nearly as much today as we have for thousands of years. Rarely, if ever, do we make any significant physical effort at all.

So how does this way of thinking affect our anatomy, physiology, psychology, and ultimately our health? Were we built to be physically inactive?

Our anatomy and physiology suggest that despite our sedentary lifestyles and bad eating habits during the last five decades or more, we are not any different from our ancestors. To be more precise, we are identical to the people who lived some 50.000 years ago! We still have bones and muscles of the same dimensions and structure, and our digestive, cardiovascular and other systems are identical to those of the early humans. This means that we still have the same genetic potential! So what is it that is so different?

The biggest disparity between our chronic disease-free ancestors and us is in the lifestyle each was compelled to adopt. We are less active today because nothing compels us to be active, we have to choose to be active. We don't exert nearly as much physical effort on the daily basis as our ancestors, and yet we eat much more and more frequently. We also eat different foods than those they had access to. And what have we to show for it? The health of our civilisation does not reflect the technological and scientific progress we have made in recent decades. Although we know more than ever before about the world around us, our own anatomy, physiology and psychology and although we fly space shuttles further out into the universe, we still suffer badly because of a relatively small problem: our lifestyle. We simply don't know how to live, what to eat, and what to do with our 600 different muscles!

Is it so impossible for us to acknowledge our own nature, to look at the size of our joints, the strength of our tendons and the ability of our heart to support strenuous physical exercise and realise that our bodies were made to be active? With our large skeletal systems, so many muscles and muscle groups and a blood pump the size of our fist, we were definitely not created to sit in a chair for the majority of the day. Today we regard sports and physical activity as either something fashionable or as someone else's chosen occupation. But proper physical engagement is not a luxury, it is a basic requirement of our everyday lives. Our physical mechanism has to be utilized in a proper and efficient way. We need to engage our full biomechanical capacity and expose every joint and muscle to the motion and effort they were created for. Only then will our bodies react positively and respond with greater health and vigour. Not a single part of the system should be neglected, because if it is, it will backfire, provoking a destructive chain reaction.

Direct and efficient physical engagement will set off natural instincts that manifest themselves in a healthy appetite for real and truly beneficial food. With regular physical exertion, proper nutrition comes spontaneously. If we look at what our bodies crave after physical exertion, we discover that we crave the very food that humans had consumed for thousands of years, the food that helped us stay away from the biggest killers of our time - the self-inflicted chronic disease.

As we are no longer engaged in the permanent struggle of the hunter/gatherer lifestyle which demanded extreme physical and mental effort, in the 21st century we must make efforts to adapt to our new lifestyle as best we can. With that in mind, we can single out one physical activity that simulates our generic lifestyle better that any other - resistance training. While we may be engaged enough mentally, physically we are not meeting our natural needs. All of our body systems have to be engaged up to a certain level and work in synergy in order for the whole system to function optimally. Our physical capabilities will deteriorate unless they are regularly and adequately engaged, as will our intellectual and mental abilities. But why is resistance training so superior to other forms of physical engagement such as games and sports, which are preferred by many people? While most of the sports we engage in activate the cardiovascular and respiratory systems to a certain de- gree and involve some of the body's muscles, none of them stress the muscular system as a whole. Other activities do not engage the totality of joints and connective tissues, heart and respira- tory system, hormonal and digestive system, and the whole body in the same way that resistance training does. Only resistance training engages our joints to their full rotational capabilities and ensures that the muscles perform their full concentric and eccentric contractions with maximum effort, while exerting the hormonal system sufficiently to produce a positive response.

There is a long list of unique benefits of resistance training. By strengthening the muscular system, resistance training strengthens the skeletal system that carries those muscles. Bones retain more calcium and become stronger in order to support larger and more active muscles. Ligaments that hold the joints together also become stronger and this enables them to last longer and allow fuller movements, which is the best prevention for common joint injuries that typically decrease mobility in people today. And it is well established that lack of mobility shortens the life-span. Muscular and skeletal strengthening together enable the individual to benefit from better posture and mobility, and greater agility. By engaging the muscular system optimally through resistance training, the cardiovascular and respiratory systems will also improve since they function as support for the muscular system. Stimulated by deep breathing, the lymphatic system will also respond positively in order to help eliminate the by-products of a more efficient metabolism. Active and regular practice of resistance training greatly improves the digestive system. Food is digested better, absorption of the essential nutrients increases and the elimination of the by-products and toxins in the body speeds up. A sufficiently active lifestyle and proper nutrition provide a foundation for an extremely strong immune system that will defend the body from infections and diseases that afflict us frequently in our modern lives. Incorporated into a healthy lifestyle, resistance training enables us to achieve the maximum potential of our generous genetic heritage, to a degree that our ancestors have never known.

Resistance training is also known as weight training or strength training. Modern technology allows us to use different types of training equipment, not just free weights, to increase the effectiveness of resistance training. Resistance training facilities today have state-of-the-art exercise equipment that satisfies the strictest criteria. We can exercise every single part of the body with full biomechanical action as part of a total body training regime, without neglecting a single muscle, joint or ligament. Through resistance training we can optimally engage our physical body while at the same time strengthening and improving our mental state. Anyone who has ever exercised with weights is familiar with a feeling of well-being and fulfilment that occurs during and after a training session. With proper technique, people regularly manage to reduce the effects of every-day stress and improve their self-confidence. As we get more energised, motivated and feel more positive about life in general, our heath and general appearance also start to be positively affected. And there is no magic to it - it is in our nature to want to be strong, healthy, productive and happy. A positive response is almost immediate – resistance training, properly applied, is the best way to benefit in all these areas in record time.

Life is all about strength. Weakness is a denial of life. We don't have to look further than the natural world around us for the confirmation of this. Fortune does not favour the weak. Physical and mental strength are the main prerequisites of a meaningful life. However, strength is not something that we can take for granted; strength has to be earned through living the right lifestyle. The moment you start thinking about improvement in any field of life, you start thinking about increasing the efficiency of your own existence. So the best starting point has to be achieving your full physical, mental and intellectual strength.

Benefits of Resistance Training

The beneficial effects of resistance training on human physical and mental condition and overall performance are well established. Resistance training engages the human body optimally. Provoking a full response in all the bodily systems brings them into a perfect balance which results in optimal health and strength. Being stronger and healthier we work better, we feel better about others and ourselves, and we perform better in other sports. It is not surprising that athletes from all the sport disciplines, after discovering its many benefits, increasingly engage in strength training.

Let's now summarise the benefits that emerge from the active engagement in resistance or strength training. The list is very long, so we shall list only those we consider to be the most significant:

Increased metabolic rate – strength training increases the body's metabolic rate, resulting in a higher expenditure of calories during resting times. This is the most important factor when it comes to fat loss. The increased metabolic ability can last up to 48 hours after high-intensity training. After a one-hour session of low-intensity, long-duration aerobic-style activity, the increased metabolic rate lasts for no more that 30 minutes.

Increased or normalised bone density – inactivity expedites the aging process, leading to a decrease in bone density causing brittleness of the bones. Weight training is the best way to increase bone density and prevent osteoporosis. Stronger and bigger muscles create the demand for higher calcium concentration in bones and faster repair of bone cells, leading automatically to stronger bones.

Increased lean-muscle mass, muscle strength, power and endurance – everyone benefits by being stronger. We can work harder, play more and we can be more productive and effective in all our endeavours, from hobbies to work-related tasks.

Decreased risk of cardiovascular disease – lowered blood pressure and decreased cholesterol levels, strengthening of the heart and improved blood circulation are benefits of strength training that directly affect our cardiovascular health.

Increased production of testosterone and growth hormone – high-intensity weight training directly stimulates the optimal production of the two most important hormones which control our physical and mental performance.

Improved glucose tolerance and insulin sensitivity – weight training can prevent diabetes by increasing the insulin sensitivity of body cells. This ultimately leads to a decrease in insulin production and optimal absorption of glucose and amino acids into cells with minimum insulin.

<u>Lower risk of cancer</u> – Regular physical activity is associated with a decreased risk of colon cancer.

<u>Better state of mind</u> – Physical activity appears to relieve symptoms of depression and anxiety and improve mood.

<u>Injury prevention</u> – The best way to prevent injuries to muscles, joints and connective tissues is to strengthen them through intense weight training.

<u>Improved balance, flexibility, mobility and stability</u> – Stronger muscles, bones, joints and connective tissues enable us to achieve all these through strength training.

<u>Rehabilitation and recovery</u> – One of the best ways to heal many types of injuries is to strengthen the muscles surrounding the injured area. The stronger your muscles, the quicker the healing process.

<u>Enhanced performance in sports or exercise</u> – No matter what your favourite sport or physical activity is, with the proper strength-training programme your performance can be dramatically improved.

<u>Feeling better and looking better</u> – Stronger muscles and joints have a dramatic impact on posture, and leaner and fitter muscles make everyone feel better about their appearance. Improved

self-esteem and increased self-confidence are direct outcomes of high-intensity weight training.

You are in Control

Being in control of our lives is a goal that everyone fights for. Being in control is being able to understand yourself, set goals and choose a direction; being able to find and select good information that is pertinent to you and your journey. It also means being motivated and confident enough to make the move, to take action required for any achievement. Accomplishing all this means that you are controlling your existence to a high degree. Achieving the results your expect is the best proof possible that you are managing to control yourself with great success. But achieving the desired goals in life is not an easy process, something that will happen just by reading manuals and books and hoping for the best.

One of the problems that often gets in the way is the amount of responsibility one has to take on. There is no success unless it carries a great deal of responsibility with it – first of all to yourself and then towards others. Often perceived as an excessive burden, responsibility deters many people from making decisions, making a move, and taking the risk of leaving their comfort zone and reaching for something higher, better, and more fertile. Many of us deny ourselves improvement simply because we fear responsibility. Once responsibility comes to be viewed as a burden and nothing more, such denial is unfortunately to be expected.

But responsibility can also be understood as enriching our lives, something that gives more substance to our existence. Once you become responsible towards yourself you will become better prepared to act correctly towards others. If you don't start by endowing yourself with more knowledge and understanding you will never be able to relate successfully to those around you. Taking responsibility as a continuous fulfilment of practical and fundamental principles of life is the best guarantee that one can live and offer others around them a good quality of life.

Analysing our own lifestyle and identifying areas that need improvement are the first steps in achieving a healthy and productive way of life, with optimal life qualities. Starting with finding the right information to help us achieve our goals, we can move on to selecting the direction in which to apply our willpower to guide us towards them.

The different areas of life should always be considered as a part of the total life engagement, and as such should be equally valued and treated. Our work, relationships, family, friendships, our intellectual and physical development and other areas of life, all are of great importance to us. From time to time we have to assign priority to one or another area in order to keep the balance in terms of quality and importance. No single area should be favoured over another. Finding the right information is a significant step in our quest for control and for a life free of misunderstanding, confusion and inaccuracy.

For the right things to start happening we have to be motivated and dedicated to our cause. Strong motivation starts with the right information which always boosts confidence. Great self-confidence grows only from the fertile soil of knowledge. Knowledge is the fountain of confidence. Together with motivation, it is a necessary prerequisites for action.

It is difficult to imagine a situation where an individual has a great deal of motivation but doesn't know what to do with it. Being sure that your task is achievable because you acquired the right information about it is the best seed for developing strong motivation.

Information and motivation alone, however, are not enough. To achieve your goals you also have to take action. Pouring your intellectual and mental powers into action is the only way to really move towards betterment. Action needs courage, and knowing what to do and how to act should eliminate the fear of failure. Insecurity and fear of failure usually come from a lack of information, or the incorrect information. Once you are equipped with the right knowledge and highly motivated, you will make the move into something new far more easily.

With the right information, motivation, targeted goals and uncompromised action, you will be on the way to self-improvement in all areas of you life. You can improve as a student, parent, friend or a professional and your continuous change towards improvement will become your new way of life, your healthiest habit.

Being in control of your life, your decisions and actions, means constantly working on yourself, persistently learning and steadily improving. Never look for the final stage of your self-improvement or the state of absolute perfection. There will never be one. It is the process itself that brings results. Knowing that you are able to identify what the right thing to do is; doing it with all your capacity and getting the expected results in the process, are all positive things that put you in charge of yourself. Once on the right track, not only will you be doing well for yourself, but you will be able to help the people around you. Once you are in a position to have knowledge, motivation and positive results, you will become more capable of transferring your experiences to others.

There are two particular themes that I would like to highlight once again because most of us simply neglect these two areas of our lives, which in the end costs us dearly. As we have demonstrated, our physical body is the prerequisite for all other forms of our existence. In order to optimise our intellectual, moral and spiritual life, to be good professionals, friends, parents and more, we have to live. Not just to live, we need to live healthily. If we neglect ourselves we will cause self-inflicted diseases that will not help us in optimising our chances for improvement. To achieve that healthy and fruitful existence, we have to engage in healthy nutrition and effective physical activity.

These two areas of healthy nutrition and effective physical activity are the most neglected areas of people's lives, but also the

areas most underestimated and ignored by life coaches and motivational speakers practicing today. Overwhelmed by their great
cause, they are consistently forgetting the basic rudiments of
healthy and productive life. Either through their lack of knowledge or personal experience, these areas are left for individuals to
discover for themselves.

After getting the right information about healthy eating and effective fitness, you will be in control of your physical existence.
Knowing that a healthy body provides the ideal environment for a
healthy mind, you can be fully confident that your starting position guarantees the most successful outcome – a healthy and balanced lifestyle with all the benefits that come with it.

Viewing your body as a temple, as the only place you have to
live in, makes you do everything in your power to manage your
health and strength and continue to live a dignified life. Being
in control of yourself, by achieving deep understanding of the
world around you and your inner being, you will make the right
choices in selecting the food that will support and fuel your life
and choose the exercise that will maintain your metabolism to its
optimal efficiency.

Once you find yourself on the right path, you will not allow ignorance and lack of knowledge to steer you in the wrong direction,
you will reject foods that steadily poison your body and your mind
and prevent you from experiencing the fantastic feeling of being

healthy, supple and strong. Being inactive and weak will never again be an option for you, as inactivity and self-inflicted loss of strength are totally incompatible with the basic notion of life.

Being in control means that you will no longer be plagued by doubts about setting goals, selecting information, generating motivation, undertaking the right action, selecting the right food or making yourself physically active in a way that will be of the maximum benefit to your anatomy. Being in control of your life gives you a chance to get the most out of what you are, move in whichever direction you want and be who you want to be.

Also from Nash Jocic:

More Books:

"The Ultimate Nutrition"

"Weight Training for Men"

"Fat Loss"

DVDs:

7 Training DVDs for Men

4 Training DVDs for Women

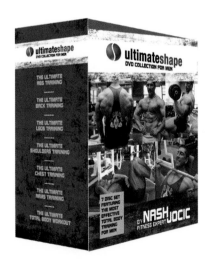 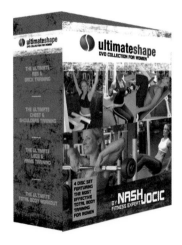

For more info see: www.ultimateshape.com